Overweight Child

How To Help Obese Children Lose Weight Fast And Become Healthy, Energetic, Confident, Successful And Happy

CRISTINA ABATE

Disclaimer

The information is of a general nature and does not take into account your personal situation. The information presented is for educational purposes only. The author will not bear any responsibility or liability for any action taken by any person, persons or organization on the purported basis of the information contained in this book and any supporting material. References to other information, websites or events should not be understood as an endorsement of such information, website or events. Every effort has been made to ensure that this book is free from errors or omissions. However, the author shall not accept responsibility for injury, loss or damage occasioned to any person acting or refraining from action as a result of material in this book whether or not such injury, loss or damage is in any way due to any negligent act or omission, breach of duty or default on the part of the author.

CONTENTS

INTRODUCTION

I want to thank you and congratulate you for buying this book, **"Overweight Child"**.

This book contains proven steps and strategies on how to help obese children lose weight fast and become healthy, energetic, confident, successful and happy.

For example, in this book we encourage family meal times to be a pleasant experience. Providing low-fat wholesome food for the entire family encourages healthier eating habits for everyone, not only for your overweight child.

This way you are not centering your overweight child out making them feel segregated from the rest of the family but instead feel like an important and loved part of the family unit.

Thanks again for purchasing this book, I hope you enjoy it!

1

DEALING WITH AND UNDERSTANDING CHILDHOOD OBESITY

As a parent you naturally worry about your child and their safety and well-being but if your child is suffering from childhood obesity this will just add to your worry and understandably so.

The National Institute of Health has released statistics recently about our overweight children.

14 industrialized countries involved in this study showed children from the United States were the most likely to be overweight.

Boys of the age of 13 were 12.6% overweight in the US

Girls of the age 13 were 10.8% overweight in the US

The number increases with the 15 year olds – 13.9% of boys are overweight and 15.1% of girls are overweight

We have a problem on our hands because obese children usually become obese adults. The numbers you just read sound scary but you can do something to help your overweight child.

First and foremost you need to educate yourselves as parents of an overweight child and learn what the dangers are that are associated with childhood obesity such as the following:

Sleep Disorders
Trouble with Bones and Joints
Low Self-Esteem
Depression
Increased Risk of High Blood Pressure
Increased Risk of Type 2 Diabetes

Your overweight child will not only be facing health problems but also psychological consequences as well.

There is a high chance that they are being teased or bullied by other kids due to their weight.

Once you learn and understand some of the causes of childhood obesity this knowledge can help you to start making better decisions for you and your family.

Genetics.

Children that have obese parents have a much higher chance of becoming obese children.

Diet.

Eating too much fast food not eating enough healthy home cooked meals. Children are drinking way too much sugary filled drinks such as sodas. Children get a large amount of added sugars in their diets from sugary drinks.

Physical Inactivity.

Many experts say that physical inactivity is the major cause of childhood obesity. Children are spending hours at a time sitting in front of video, TV, computer screens getting no physical exercise.

Environment.

Kids are over exposed to commercials always trying to sell all kinds of junk foods. Our schools are only offering on average 2.1 PE classes a week which adds up to an insufficient amount of exercise around 68.7 minutes a week.

Visit Child's Doctor.

Take your child to their doctor to have them examined to see if the doctor diagnosis them with childhood obesity or not. It is best to have your child checked by a physician and get a medical diagnosis.

.

2

PSYCHOSOCIAL ASPECTS OF CHILDHOOD OBESITY

Families that are receiving counseling on making sure they understand the importance of providing adequate healthy meals and physical activity for the children in the family especially one that is suffering from childhood obesity must make a serious effort to improve the lifestyle of the family.

If you are parents of an overweight child that feel lost in what to do to help your child perhaps seeking counseling from clinicians can help you as parents to learn ways to help provide physical activities, emotional support for your child and nutritional food to help bring your child to a healthier weight.

You can also learn about the psychosocial factors that can be contributing to your child's weight problem. They could be suffering from low self-esteem, depression, weight bias, bullying. They could be dealing with experiences that are making it difficult for them to achieve a healthy outcome. Clinicians can try and identify what the underlying stressors are and try and implement proper counseling to help resolve these issues.

By helping to promote healthy living from a clinical setting it is helping to guide families towards a healthier lifestyle. Besides addressing the physical and nutritional issues the parents must also become aware of the psychosocial factors that are contributing to their child's obesity.

Children that have depression, low self-esteem, bullying and weight bias will find it more difficult to manage their weight. Clinicians can help families to try and reach goals that are realistic and appropriate.

Psychosocial Contributors to Obesity.

There are psychosocial contributors to obesity such as stressors that may trigger emotional eating in a child. If a child is suffering from neglect or malnutrition with limited supervision of child these could be triggers that cause the child to partake in emotional eating. Children that are stressed are more prone to emotional or overeating.

This is a form of eating that is to give one's self some comfort or to make one's self less attractive. Common stressors in children that lead to overeating are when parents are divorcing, separating or fighting all the time in front of the child, physical and mental abuse, bullying and living in foster care.

Poor sleeping habits can start in a child due to chronic stress. Child may show signs of fatigue or reluctance to get involved with any physical activities at school or at home. The lack of sleep is a known risk factor for obesity. The immune system can be negatively affected by stress it can increase the risk of viral upper respiratory infections.

Psychological Affects of Childhood Obesity.

Children that suffer from childhood obesity will not only have higher health risks of developing type 2 diabetes, high cholesterol, high blood pressure, and sleeping problems but will likely have a hard time with their emotions as well.

Researchers have found that it doesn't matter what your age is but that carrying around extra weight is going to have its psychological consequences.

When living as a member of a stigmatized group it can be very stressful causing depression, anxiety and loneliness for your child. These negative feelings can have a great impact on all aspects of your child's life such as academic performance.

Playground: Tough Spot to be for Overweight Children.

The playground is a place where much of the bullying and teasing takes place which the overweight children get the most of it. Name calling can really grate on a child's self-esteem.

Overweight children internalize what others feedback on them is such as calling them fat, no good and telling them no one wants to be their friend. This type of abuse contributes towards anxiety and depression.

It is estimated that rates of depression are 20 percent in overweight children. Depression occurs due to being overweight and constantly getting teased and bullied about it from other children.

Kids that are suffering from depression are more likely to gain weight than to participate in exercise. Studies have shown that children who have been bullied try to avoid places they were getting bullied such as gym class and sports fields. Bullied kids tend to be more depressed, lonely and anxious.

Problems Arise Early.

Though understanding an overweight school child gaining more weight due to their avoiding physical activity it doesn't explain the weight gain of very young children from age 2 as early as 3 months showing early signs of obesity. If this extra weight comes early in life so will the psychological consequences. By the time overweight children are in third grade they already see themselves as disliked or unpopular.

Children that suffer from childhood obesity are more likely to be lonely, sad, and worry more than children who don't have a weight problem. As they get older these feelings just get worse.

3

WHAT CAN PARENTS DO?

Parents that want to help their child slim down must also work at keeping their child's self-esteem intact.

Constant nagging at a child about their weight is not going to see a positive outcome.

But either will letting your child eat whatever they want.

Parents should let their child know that they are concerned about their child's health not how they look.

Getting an overweight child to get out and exercise will help to build their self-esteem in addition to the physical health benefits. By making sure that your child gets 40 minutes of exercise a day will help to lessen depression and make them feel better about themselves.

Tips for Parents.

1) Try and create an environment where your child can learn to feel good about themselves. Introduce them to hobbies, sports, neighborhood activities. Encourage them to pursue things that they enjoy or are interested in. Help them to recognize that by taking care of their body it can allow them to do what they would like to do.

2) Help your child learn how to deal with bullying and teasing. You could role play showing them how to avoid reacting to unkind words and actions and just walking away. Teach them to make positive "I message" such as "I am ignoring these mean words because they are not true."

3) Make sure to turn off the TV during family meal time sit down and have a family meal discussing the day's events with your child.

Parents Get Blamed for Childhood Obesity.

Studies have shown that children tend to eat what their parents eat. Suggestions have been made that there is a parental contribution to the growing obesity problem in young children.

Researchers have found that if parents are eating 4-5 pieces of servings of fruit and vegetables a day then so are their children. If parents are eating a lot of fast foods and sodas the children are eating the same.

Good dieting habits start at home, if parents are eating poorly chances are the children will be too.

A study done in California found that:

30 percent of teenagers are overweight.
Teens that parents drink soda are 40 percent more likely to drink soda too than teens that parents don't drink soda.
Teens that parent's eat 4-5 servings of fruit and vegetables a day are 16 percent more likely to do the same then teens whose parents don't eat five servings a day.
Nearly half of teens (48) percent whose parents drink soda everyday eat fast foods at least once a day only 39 percent of teens eat fast foods whose parents do not drink soda.

The research points towards parents being somewhat responsible for teen obesity and helping to resolve it will also start with the parents. While parents are the primary role models for their children their behavior can have a positive or a negative influence on their children's health. It is also essential to start to find ways to help low-income communities get access to fruits and vegetables and other healthy foods.

Girls vs. Boys.

Our children are constantly bombarded with images of the perfect bodies through different media sources.

For girls it is often to be skinny and to diet and exercise.

For boys the message tends to be that he should bulk up get into weight lifting and build up his muscles. This can lead to use of dietary supplements and steroids that can be harmful.

Girls tend to be at higher risk of developing eating disorders due to the pressures of society pressuring them to be skinny.

Society tends to have a wider-range of acceptable body images for boys. But they too are also susceptible to developing eating disorders all in the hopes of getting the perfect body that society pressures them to have if they want to be an accepted part of society.

.

4

PLANNING A HEALTHY DIET FOR THE WHOLE FAMILY

You must discuss your plans of putting the whole family on a diet with your spouse or partner explaining that it is to help and support your overweight child in hopefully losing some weight without them getting centered out and feeling segregated from the rest of the family.

Your plan to make it a family diet will not only make your overweight child feel more comfortable but also it will benefit the whole family's health by trying to live a healthier lifestyle taking up this challenge as a family helping to support one another building closer relationships will make you stronger as a family.

Your overweight child is probably already suffering from being isolated at school due to their childhood obesity.

Overweight children tend to become withdrawn trying to avoid being bullied by other children who may tease them about their weight.

Do not let your overweight child know that you are putting the family on a diet to help them they could end up feeling resentment towards you and become more withdrawn.

Make a point of letting them think that this is not about them but about getting the whole family healthy. Make sure to agree to stick with the eating plan that you decide to go with you must make sure to back your spouse up on the decisions on what foods will be eaten when.

Decide together when electronic games or video games etc. are allowed and for what period of time, organizing family weekend outings such as going to the zoo or local park to play some ball. Get children involved in helping to decide what the family activity will be on the weekend.

You as parents must show by example your children look up to you for guidance. Setting good eating habits and getting daily exercise is setting good examples for your children.

Before you go shopping plan out the meals for the week writing down all that you need to make them on your shopping list. Try to stick to your shopping list as much as possible because if it is not on your weekly menu list it is not something you really need. Try and be firm with your children if they are trying to get you to buy unhealthy foods you must be firm and say no but offer some healthy alternatives to them to choose from.

Sometimes when you make a start date for a diet it helps to make it more official and real when you put it on the family calendar announcing to the family when the family diet will begin. This gives everyone in the family a chance to prepare themselves for the diet challenge ahead.

When you choose a start date it is making a commitment to following through with starting the family diet challenge. Discuss your thoughts of putting the whole family on a healthier daily diet plan and ask their thoughts on it. Explain to them how important it is to you that the family starts eating and living a healthier lifestyle.

Let them know that as a parent you want to provide the best for your children starting with the basics of healthy food choices. Once your family understands why you are doing this diet challenge they will more than likely want to help support you in it.

5

REDUCING ADDED SUGARS IN YOUR FAMILY'S DIET

As parents you must try and make the healthy food decisions perhaps having one night on the weekend where you have a fun meal such as pizza you could make Saturday night pizza and movie night for the entire family.

Try making homemade pizza getting your children involved in preparing the pizza using whole wheat dough along with some healthy fun toppings. Try and get your child that is overweight involved allowing them to help you to prepare meals will help to teach them to prepare healthier meal choices.

Also get them involved in preparing sweet treats that have no added sugars but still will satisfy the sweet tooth that big and little kids alike have of all ages. By making healthy sweets with your overweight child you are teaching them that they can still have fun sweet foods as part of a healthy diet.

By preparing meals and doing some baking together will give you a chance to make your bonds stronger with your family members especially your overweight child by drawing them out of seclusion to help you in the kitchen. They will feel proud of their culinary skills at moments when a dish that they helped prepare is getting rave reviews from the rest of the family members.

This is a great way to help build your overweight child's self-confidence up as well as help build skills that they can use for the rest of their life.

Below are a few suggestions of healthy snacks, lunches and dinners that you may want to try if you are looking for some healthy meal ideas.

.

6

HEALTHY SNACK SUGGESTIONS

1) No-sugar added applesauce sprinkle with cinnamon and raisins on top

2) Cubed Pineapple with low-fat cottage cheese

3) Air-popped light popcorn

4) Homemade Trail Mix use some favorite nuts, dried fruits, cereals, great for putting in individual bags using as snacks at school or work

5) Granola Bars

6) Spread peanut-butter on apple slices then top with coconut and raisins.

7) Smoothies – can be a great meal replacement get creative adding many different combinations of fruit and vegetables in your smoothies. Allow your children to help choose what to add in their smoothies

8) Cheerios topped with fruit such as bananas or berries with some low-fat milk

9) Whole wheat pita bread with some almond butter

10) Homemade potato fries using sweet potatoes drizzle with extra virgin olive oil and bake in the oven at 325 for about 30 minutes flipping halfway through.

11) Half a bagel with smoked salmon on top

12) Cup of veggie soup

13) Celery sticks with raisins and peanut-butter on top

14) Hard boiled eggs

15) Plain yogurt add some fresh fruit

16) Grapes in a bag for snack

17) Piece of fruit

18) Vegetable sticks with low-fat dip

19) Handful of nuts

20) Sugar-free Muffin with blueberries

Sugar Free Deserts.

1) Baked apples done in the microwave
Prep Time: 5 minutes
Cook Time: 5 minutes

Directions:
Core the apples then fill middle with fruit and nuts of your choice then sprinkle outside with Stevia for baking add cinnamon too then bake for 5 minutes let stand for 5 minutes before you serve.

2) Fruit Dip:
Prep Time: 15 minutes
Serving: 4
Ingredients:
1 teaspoon of grated orange peel
1 tablespoon of fresh orange juice
3 ounces of light plain yogurt
4 ounces of fat-free cream cheese

Directions:
Let the cream cheese soften then add remaining ingredients to it mix well with an electric blender store in covered container. Then serve with fresh pieces of fruit works great at a party offering a healthy and tasty snack to your guests.

3) Grilled Blueberry or Strawberry Sandwich:
Prep Time: 2 minutes
Cook Time: 5 minutes
Number of servings: 2
Ingredients:
1 whole wheat pita bread
1 cup of blueberries or strawberries mashed with a bit of stevia
3 tablespoons of low-fat cream cheese

Directions:
Cut the pita opening the pocket then combine cream cheese with other ingredients then spread into the pocket close and grill on both sides with a non-stick skillet.

Lunch Suggestions:

1) Greek Salad

2) Turkey on whole wheat pita with thin slice of Swiss cheese, balsamic dressing and spinach

3) Ham & Cheese sandwich on dark rye bread served with dill pickles on the side

4) Tomato soup with 4 whole wheat crackers and cheese

5) Vegetable soup with 4 whole wheat crackers and cheese

6) Garden salad with yogurt and fresh fruit pieces

7) BLT on dark rye bread with garden salad

8) Salmon on whole wheat pita with spinach

9) Broccoli soup with 4 whole wheat crackers and cheese

10) Ham & Cheese omelet

Dinner Suggestions:

1) Pork chops with non-added sugar applesauce on top bake in oven at 325 for 30 minutes with baked potato and serve with carrots and peas

2) Tuna Casserole

3) Beef Stew

4) Chili

5) Stir Fry using oriental veggies and cubed chicken breast brown chicken then add veggies serve with brown rice

6) Balsa Fish served with brown rice and asparagus

7) Steak & Shrimp barbequed serve with salad of your choice

8) Whole wheat pasta with vegetarian spaghetti sauce

9) Barbequed Salmon Steak with fresh dill and lemon serve with brown rice and Brussel sprouts

10) Skinless Chicken Breast with mushroom sauce serve with brown rice and steamed asparagus

To help you further look for ideas for healthy foods below is a great link to an Australian website that is based out of Melbourne offering wonderful sugar free snacks and desert recipes geared to appeal to kids.

I am sure you will find some great fun recipes there that you can try with your child; you will both benefit greatly from this experience of learning how to make healthy fun sweet treats. Of course the other members of your family will also benefit from these yummy healthy treats too!

http://www.sugarfreekids.com.au/

7

GETTING YOUR CHILD INVOLVED IN LOW-IMPACT EXERCISE

Often with overweight children they tend to shy away from being involved in team sports due to the bullying they must endure from other children.

Many overweight children become loners isolating themselves from others including family.

Try and find an activity that your child shows an interest in then make an effort to get them involved in some kind of daily activity that will give them some physical exercise.

Four Legged Friend for Your Child.

If you do not have a dog this could be a good companion for your child and will encourage your child to play with it and take it for walks this will result in your overweight child also getting some physical exercise.

Make sure before you agree to get your child a dog that you lay some ground rules down those being that the child must walk the dog every day after school and feed and care for the dog and clean up after it.

If your child does not properly care for the dog make sure that you tell them that the dog will be given away. This is just to make sure that you make your child realize how important it is that they make sure to take proper care of their pet. By making them responsible for their pet it builds up their self-confidence in knowing they are capable of taking care of another living being.

They may even meet new friends while walking their dog because often people will stop dog owners to ask about their dog and if they can pet them etc. Friendships could even develop from these interactions for your child maybe becoming friends with a fellow dog lover.

A dog will show your child unconditional love as a dog does not care if it's owner is overweight it will love it's owner no matter what they look like.

The dog has been called "man's best friend" due to the love and loyalty they show towards their owners. I am sure your child will feel delighted to see their tail wagging friend waiting at the door to greet them after a hard day at school.

Perhaps on the weekends the whole family can go for walks on trails getting everybody out in the fresh air getting some good low-impact exercise and spending some quality time with the whole family including the four-legged member!

Rollerblading.

This is a fun low-impact form of exercise that you and your overweight child or another sibling could do together. It gets your child outside in the fresh air and having some fun while getting some much needed exercise at the same time.

When something is fun to do it does not seem like exercise your child will want to do it again just for the fun of it nothing more!

Swimming.

This is another fun form of low-impact exercise that most children love to do.

You could take your child to the local pool for a swim together if you do not own a pool perhaps even join a child parent exercise class that involves dancing in the water to music.

This could be a really fun thing to do together that will also provide you both with a full body workout.

The water will provide extra resistance helping your muscles to get more of a challenging workout but not putting any added stress on your joints. Doing a workout in the water will improve your core, legs, arms as well as your cardiovascular fitness.

This is a form of exercise that could benefit the whole family. When you go on holidays why not take your family camping at a lake where you can all swim and perhaps do some canoeing another great form of exercise.

Family Bike Rides.

You should consider getting a bike rack for your family vehicle so that you can travel to different areas to do some family bike rides.

When you go on holiday if you have a bike rack you can take your bikes along on your camping trip. This is a good form of exercise that you can encourage your overweight child to do by joining them on a bike ride. Your children enjoy spending time with you so spending that time wisely by doing an activity with them that is beneficial to both of you is a smart idea.

Stop Driving Everywhere.

Instead of jumping in your car every time you need to go somewhere start trying to walk or ride your bikes more often. Say for example you want to go to the library with your child instead of driving there take a walk to the library or a bike ride.

All these little changes in your lifestyle will make a positive difference in many ways for you and your overweight child.

Eventually by continuing with doing daily exercise of some sort you will start to notice your child will be improving both inside and outside.

Once they have been eating healthier and getting some form of regular physical exercise for awhile you will see your child start to bloom into a healthier happier child living a better quality of life compared to their past unhealthy lifestyle.

Not only will your child blossom into a healthier person but your family as a whole will be blossoming from living a healthier lifestyle.

Community Events.

Find out what is going on in your community as far as family events or activities offered to the children of your community perhaps you can find something that interests your child that you may even be able to participate in together or do as a family.

Try and find an after school activity to join your child in that will get them out of the house and interacting with others. Maybe there is a parent child cooking class being offered that you and your child could join together to help teach you both how to prepare healthy meals.

CONCLUSION

Thank you again for purchasing this book!

I hope this book was able to help get your obese child to lose weight fast and become healthy, energetic, confident, successful and happy.

I appreciate you for taking the time out of your day or evening to read this book, and if you have an extra second, I would love to hear what you think about this book by leaving a review on Amazon. I would greatly appreciate it!

Go to http://amzn.to/1y8iyNA

If the links do not work, for whatever reason, you can simply search for the title "Overweight Child" on the Amazon website.

Thank you again, and I wish you nothing but the best!

Cristina Abate

HERE IS A BOOK I RECOMMEND CALLED
"FOLLOW YOUR OWN PATH"

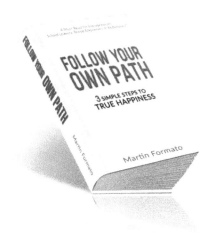

This is the coolest book I have ever read and by purchasing a copy you put another copy into the hands of someone less fortunate as the author's mission which is to inspire people to do what they love that also contributes to humanity. That is a win/win/win.

Who Is This Book For?

This book is for anyone who is hungry.

Anyone who wants more out of life.

Anyone who knows that they have more to give, share and experience.

Anyone who feels deep down, in their heart, that they are here for a reason.

It's a book for people who feel stuck, lost, depressed or even suicidal.

In particular, it's for, entrepreneurs who are struggling, school leavers who are lost, employees who are bored or in a job they hate and redundees who feel discarded.

Today, more than ever in history, people need more direction and less information.

This book will put you on the right path, YOUR PATH.

Who Is This Book NOT For?

You should not get this book until you are certain that you truly wish to change your life and you are 100 percent committed to it.

Ask yourself these 2 questions:

1. Do I want to make a change voluntarily, completely of my own choice?
2. Do I really want to change my life?

If you cannot honestly say "Yes" without hesitation to both questions, then it is better that you wait until you are serious about changing your life.

As one monk famously said "We want only warriors… victims need not apply".

Go to: http://amzn.to/2kQC9CK

If the links do not work, for whatever reason, you can simply search for the title "Follow Your Own Path" on the Amazon website.

CONTENTS FROM THE BOOK
"FOLLOW YOUR OWN PATH"

STEP 3: GIVE YOUR PASSION TO THE WORLD

Go to http://amzn.to/2kQC9CK

If the links do not work, for whatever reason, you can simply search for the title "Follow Your Own Path" on the Amazon website.

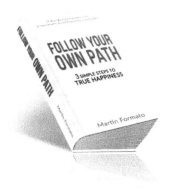

BONUS: FREE BOOK

Go to the website at www.DoingWorkThatMatters.com and enter your email address to get the FREE book "**Find Your Gift, Passion and Purpose**".

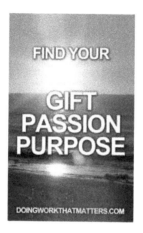

Once you register you will be sent FREE information that will further help you create a life you love.

All you have to do is enter your email address to get instant access.

This information will help you get more out of your life – to be able to reach your goals, have more motivation, be at your best, and live the life you have always dreamed of.

New resources are continually added, which you will be notified of as a subscriber. These will help you live your life to the fullest!

CPSIA information can be obtained
at www.ICGtesting.com
Printed in the USA
LVHW011102120922
728117LV00001B/203